Intermittent Fasting for Busy Women

Reach your Weight Loss Goals While Managing your Busy Schedule

Table of Contents

Introduction

It is true that we are living in a busy world. To some of us, the twenty-four hours are somewhat insufficient to carry out everything we have to do in a day. Nowadays, most people find time as the major limiting factor to various commitments. Due to the time factor, people forget good habits including healthy diets. Women, especially, spend so much time on their personal, work, and family issues that they forget to follow good dietary habits. In fact, studies show that a large percentage of women use their time attending to family issues. Making meals for the family makes it impossible for them to follow recommended diet plans. This can be attributed to the fact that women tend to eat what they have just prepared for their family. In many cases, a dietary disorder is the only thing that reminds them how important it is to adhere to proper eating patterns. Being a woman means more than doing chores, looking out for your children (if you have some), going to the grocery store, and preparing meals. Taking care of your health is a personal obligation, regardless of how busy you may be. According to advice by nutritionists, keeping our bodies healthy is of paramount importance. Without proper health, we will not even be able to carry out any of our routines. We need to adopt and adhere to eating habits that are in line with standard health requirements. One of the simplest guidelines is eating a balanced diet, which we infrequently observe. Well, we are only human! However, ignorance is no defense. We should not pretend to be unaware of existing dietary information that can improve our eating patterns. One may consult a nutritionist or search online for dietary plans and tips.

There are many diet tactics that women can adopt, irrespective of their busy schedules. Among them is intermittent fasting. It is the most ideal diet plan that can help women to lose weight without spending time at the gym. Nonetheless, commitment and persistence must prevail.

Chapter One
What is Intermittent Fasting?

Intermittent fasting is a dietary plan that involves scheduled eating. This means that you eat only at specific times and completely avoid food even when you feel hungry. At first, practicing intermittent fasting may be hard to cope with. Before you get used to fasting, it is advisable to eat a snack before the indicated meal time. Usually, most people find a six- to eight-hour window as the ideal period to practice intermittent fasting.

For example, intermittent fasting may include skipping breakfast and eating later in the day, around 12:00 to 1:00 p.m. On the other hand, some people may eat a "heavy" breakfast and eat small meals throughout the day.

Notably, intermittent fasting does not in any way involve a specific diet. It is just a dieting pattern. Fasting by itself is a method and not a diet. Fasting aims at changing our lifestyle and does not have anything to do with what we eat. It is about when to eat.

How Does Intermittent Fasting Work?

Understanding how intermittent fasting works begins with understanding the distinction between the fed state and the fasted state. In the fed state, the body is able to digest and absorb food. Basically, the fed state starts after eating and continues for the next three to five hours during digestion and absorption. During this time, it is hard to burn fat because insulin levels are very high.

Afterward, the body enters a post-absorptive state where food is not processed. This period lasts for the next eight to twelve hours after the meal. At this time, the body is deemed to be in a fasted state. It is easier for the body to burn fat in a fasted state since insulin levels are low.

When in a fasted state, the body can also burn fat that is inaccessible during a fed state. This is why beginners of intermittent fasting lose a lot of body fat without changing what they eat, how much they eat, or how often they exercise. Fasting sets the body into a fat- burning state that cannot be achieved with a normal eating schedule.

Types of Intermittent Fasting

Are you considering giving intermittent fasting a try? Note that there are various options that can help you make fasting a part of your lifestyle. This section aims to elaborate on the commonest methods of intermittent fasting that can be employed by women. It is imperative to note that different methods have better results for different people. Consulting a dietician for a personalized method of intermittent fasting is crucial. Even so, one should select the method that is easiest and most comfortable to follow. Otherwise, the health benefits may be short-lived or not experienced at all. Below is detailed information about different intermittent fasting methods.

Daily Intermittent Fasting (Leangains) Method

This method was first explained by Martin Berkhan of leangains.com. He recommends that the method should be employed by gym-goers who want to lose extremely high levels of body fat and build more muscle. Basically, the method involves a sixteen-hour-fast, followed by an eight-hour eating period. However, women are advised to fast for fourteen hours each day and eat for the remaining ten hours.

Many people refer to this method as the 16/8 method. As stated above, one should restrict eating and squeeze in two or three meals within the eight to ten hours. The majority of people following this method skip breakfast and have their first meal at midday. The other meal is eaten before going to bed but not late at night.

During the fasting period, one should not consume any calories. Only calorie-free sweeteners, diet soda, black coffee, and sugar-free gum are permitted. Most followers of this method find it easiest to fast throughout the night. What and when you eat during the eating window depends on whether or not you're following any workout program. On the day you plan to exercise, definitely don't fast. Your body needs to replenish the energy used up during exercising. It is easy to follow daily intermittent fasting because it is practiced every day. With daily intermittent fasting, the only change required is specific eating times.

Pros: The major advantage of this method is that you can eat whatever you want within the "eating" window. No specific type of food is restricted. Moreover, you can eat small amounts of meals as many times as possible within the period.

Cons: On the other hand, the disadvantage to this method is flexibility in when to eat. For maximum results, the time frame for eating should be a maximum of ten hours.

Eat Stop Eat Method (Weekly Intermittent Fasting)

In this method of intermittent fasting, one should fast for twenty-four hours once or twice in a week. Brad Pilon developed this method with an aim of helping dieters to get "motivated" to eat after a long window of fasting. In other words, this method enhances hunger throughout the whole day, causing one to eat more effectively when the time comes.

During the fasting period, no food is consumed. However, you can drink calorie-free beverages. You can only go back to your usual eating patterns after the fast is over. Some people need to finish the fasting period at a normal mealtime with a big serving. Dieticians suggest that one consume a bowl of warm soup before eating to "awake" the digestive system. Hard foods may hurt the inactive digestive tract and cause inflammation, accompanied by constipation.

This method reduces overall caloric intake without limiting what one is able to eat. Incorporating short-lived workouts can improve weight loss. Note that this should be brief workouts because you do not want to lose the energy you need to sail through the next twenty-four hours (or forty-eight hours) without a meal.

Pros: This method is flexible. Beginners who may not find the method easy to cope with can simply maximize the number of hours they go without food even if it is not twenty-four hours. After the body has adjusted, one can gradually increase the fasting phase over time.

Cons: Going for twenty-four hours or more without any calories may not be easy for some people, especially for the first few weeks. In fact, the majority of dieters may struggle with going for extended periods with no food. They cite annoying symptoms such as headaches, stomachaches, fatigue, feeling cranky, or anxious. However, these are minor side effects of a lack of calories and energy in the body which diminish over time.

The Warrior Diet

This type of fasting is also called the 20/4 method. In this method, fasting becomes more intense, with twenty hours without food, allowing only a four-hour window for eating. It is most likely that only one meal can be consumed. The meal should be large enough to fill you up and adequately provide the body with necessary nutrients. Therefore, this should be a balanced diet. Mainly, this method is tailored for people who can follow strict rules.

The Warrior Diet is based on the philosophy that human beings are nocturnal eaters and are inherently programmed to eat at night. Moreover, it's suggested that the body needs nutrients for proper syncing of its circadian rhythms. The fasting phase of the Warrior Diet entails "undereating." Even as this is the case, one can have a few servings of fruits, fresh juice, or raw veggies in the course of the twenty hours. This is aimed at enhancing the nervous system to promote alertness, boost energy levels, and stimulate fat burning. In the four-hour "overeating" window, one should eat enough food to help the body recuperate. Additionally, this will promote relaxation and calm the metabolism and digestion while allowing the body to use the nutrients consumed in order to enhance repair and growth.

Nutritionists suggest that eating at night helps the body to produce hormones and burn fats during the day. According to the inventor of this fasting method, the order in which one eats specific food groups matters. One should start with veggies, proteins, and fat.

Carbohydrates should be eaten only when one feels hungry, even after eating.

Pros: Many people adopt this fasting method because it allows one to eat a few small snacks within the twenty hours. As mentioned above, one can eat some fruits or raw veggies. Many practitioners of this method report an increased rate in energy and fat loss.

Cons: The long hours of fasting are strict with snacking. This may interfere with social gatherings. Friends, relatives, and colleagues may not understand why you should not share a meal with them just because you are on a diet. Additionally, the recommended eating time may not be suitable for everyone. Who wants to wake up at night to eat? This makes it hard, especially for people who do not prefer eating at night, and for those who like eating small, consistent meals.

Alternate Day Fasting (ADF)

This method is also called the 5:2 Diet Plan. It entails severely restricting calories two days of the week and eating whatever you want the other five days. The method was invented by James Johnson with an aim of helping disciplined dieters with a specific weight loss goal. Notably, this method is different from the "Eat, Stop, Eat method" because one can eat something during the two days of fasting. An example of the alternate day fasting schedule may include Tuesday and Friday as the fasting days within a week.

Practicing alternate day fasting is all about lowering caloric intake for two days and maximizing it the other five days. This means that on low-calorie days, a diet should be one-fifth of normal caloric intake. Using an example of 2,000 calories for female dieters during the five days, four-hundred calories is the ideal amount for the two days of low-calorie intake.

To make low-calorie days easier to adopt, one may opt for shakes and smoothies. Generally, they are fortified with essential nutrients and can be sipped throughout the day as substitutes for small meals. Working out may be incorporated during the five days of high-calorie intake. It can help to burn the many calories.

Pros: This method is all about weight loss. It is best adopted by people whose sole aim is weight loss. Cutting caloric intake by twenty to thirty-five percent may see a person lose about two to three pounds per week.

Cons: While this method is very easy to follow, one can overindulge on high-calorie days. There is no specific limit in the number of calories that a dieter should eat. After all, the inventor's recommendation is to eat what one feels like during the five days.

Note that any type of intermittent fasting should be based on the guidance of a dietician. This is because there are a few factors that need to be considered before fasting. For example, your health is key to determining whether or not you should try fasting. You may be taking medication that requires you to eat a lot of food. Your doctor should have a say in the method of fasting you should adopt.

Who Should Practice Intermittent Fasting?

Nutritionists are still scratching the surface, trying to understand the role of intermittent fasting in the overall health of dieters. Intermittent fasting may work for one person and fail miserably for another. Adopting this method for weight loss should be done with the full knowledge of a dietician. It is prudent to get an expert to walk you safely through the best regimen for you. There is an unending debate about who should and should not adopt intermittent fasting. The section below aims at clearing up the matter.

Who Can Adopt Intermittent Fasting?

When it comes to intermittent fasting, there are a plethora of different methods, of varying difficulties. Considering the benefits and risks, intermittent fasting is best for people who aim to lose weight fast and permanently. It's also good for people who enjoy a wide variety of foods and do not want restrictions on some types of food. This is because intermittent fasting does not necessarily dictate restrictions but only directs people on the time of day they should eat.

Intermittent fasting may also be helpful for people who tend to have digestive problems at night. They can adopt intermittent fasting to ensure that they do not consume anything before going to sleep. This will prevent heartburn, acid reflux, and other digestive woes. Anyone wishing to experience the benefits of intermittent fasting should feel free to take up the dieting plan, but with approval by their personal doctor

Who Should Avoid Intermittent Fasting?

Even though most studies recommend intermittent fasting due to countless health benefits, it is not for everyone. For example, individuals with insulin-dependent diabetes should avoid intermittent fasting. Moreover, lactating mothers and pregnant women should not engage in intermittent fasting. This is because fasting leads to missing important nutrients which are required for the healthy growth of a baby. In both cases, a woman's health should also be prioritized.

Intermittent fasting is not ideal for amateur or professional athletes. An athlete's body depends on perfectly timed fuel before and after training sessions for performance and recovery. Therefore, they need to be able to consume food at any time of the day. It may be fatal to skip meals after exercising because your body energy needs to be replenished. One can only do that by eating.

In many cases, there are several factors that should serve as a green light for anyone intending to use intermittent fasting. As a dieter, you will be successful with intermittent fasting if:

- You have a history of strictly monitoring calorie and food intake. This simply means that you have dieted before.

- You are an experienced exerciser. This will enhance weight loss and boost muscle building.

- You are not planning to get pregnant any soon. Do not forget that intermittent fasting can have life-threatening effects on you and to the fetus.

- You are not pregnant or lactating within the period of fasting.

- You have a flexible job which allows for periods of low performance. This reduces the potential side effects of having low energy.

Chapter Two
Incorporating Fasting into your Lifestyle

Introduction

Do you want to adopt intermittent fasting but have no idea about where to start? This part of the book aims at helping you understand the simple steps necessary for incorporating fasting into your lifestyle. Even though fasting will be hard at some point, you only need to remain focused on your goals. Here are some key procedures to follow when incorporating fasting into your lifestyle.

Consult Your Dietician Before Beginning Intermittent Fasting

It is always important to seek advice from your dietician about any dietary changes you're considering. Get as much information as possible about the pros and cons of the diet. Disclose all food sensitivities you may have. Additionally, inform the dietician of any pre-existing medical conditions that you may have including diabetes, ulcers, and irritable bowel syndrome, among others. This will help the dietician to make better decisions on whether or not the diet plan in question is right for you. Do not be overlook the fact that intermittent fasting can have dramatic effects on your metabolism. Some can be fatal, especially if you ignore life-threatening symptoms. Quickly notify your dietitian about any irregularities after starting fasting.

Choose a Fasting Protocol You Want to Follow

As seen from an earlier section of this book, there are several types of intermittent fasting. As a quick review of these methods, they include Leangains, Eat, Stop, Eat, The Warrior Diet, and Alternate-Day Fasting. Of course, at the discretion of many dieters, there may be many other types of fasting. However, it may not be recommendable for a beginner to follow unverified methods of intermittent fasting. Choosing a fasting method entails evaluating your capability. For example, are you able to for over twenty-four hours without food (for the Eat, Stop, Eat) or are you just able to cut down caloric intake while eating small amounts of food (for Leangains)? This is as simple as understanding what is easiest for you.

Moderately Reduce Daily Calorie Consumption

Whichever method you chose to adopt, ensure that you decrease calorie consumption over time. This includes every mealtime. If you normally eat 2,000 to 3000 calories per day, this is an indication that you cannot cut the number instantly. It is better to reduce caloric intake gradually to avoid problems from drastically cutting calories. As a start, try not to exceed 1500 calories per day.

Afterward, try and get below 1000 calories. The journey will continue until you reach the recommended bare minimum of about four-hundred calories per day. To achieve this, customize your diet to include healthy carbs. Avoid foods that contain complex carbs and fats. Other foods to avoid include white bread and white noodles.

Create a Viable Meal Plan

A meal plan is an outline of what to eat and when to eat. You should formulate a realistic and easy-to-follow meal plan. It doesn't have to be boring, restrictive, or inconvenient. The ideal meal plan should be flexible and leave options for impromptu eating when you get an invitation for lunch or dinner with a friend. You wouldn't want to turn down the request just because you are fasting. After such a meal, you should have a personally crafted way of fasting for a longer period. While at home, ensure that you eat the right kind of foods. Avoid being too restrictive with foods you love, but do not overeat.

Tips on How to Put Fasting into Practice

Some people may find it hard to follow intermittent fasting, especially if they have no knowledge of how to put it into practice. The whole process may be simplified by learning some tips. This part of the book provides a number of tips you can use from the comfort of your home, instead of visiting a dietician.

Choose an Eating Plan That You Can Maintain

It is good to bear in mind that intermittent fasting will make you go without food for a long period of time. Typically, the order of fasting should take at least fourteen hours per day. One should select an eating plan which contains a favorable number of hours. Avoid subjecting yourself to a long fasting period that is not sustainable even for a whole week. Set an eating plan with two main meals to ensure satiety.

Do Not Dramatically Alter Your Diet

When on intermittent fasting, it is unnecessary to cut down any specific food groups. You are good to go as long as you eat a balanced and healthy diet and do not exceed 1,000 calories for the first few weeks. Ultimately, you will find yourself at the recommended trimmed calorie intake of about four-hundred to five-hundred calories. Note that it is not important to change the types of food you eat before beginning. Continue eating adequate proteins, fruits and vegetables, and moderate amounts of carbohydrates. Just concern yourself with changing your eating schedule and not the types of foods that you eat.

Set a Weight Loss Goal

The success of intermittent fasting is measured by the degree of weight loss. Most importantly, this happens by reducing daily caloric intake to allow the body to burn off fat reserves. Decreasing the number of hours you spend eating will cause you to lose weight. This will raise your metabolism and reduce the amount of inflammation in your body. Setting a weight loss goal will keep you motivated to follow your diet. For example, as a beginner, you can set a maximum intake of 1,500 calories

This should last for the first five days. Afterward, set another goal to reduce calories to 1,000 in the next five days. As the body adjusts to the gradual reduction of calories, set goals to become a better fasting dieter.

Fast During Sleeping Hours

Even as some people may find it tolerable to eat the last meal at night, it should not be very late at night. The night is deemed the most appropriate time for fasting. This is because sleeping keeps the mind off a growling stomach. In fact, it is rare to notice a rumbling stomach while you are deep asleep. In addition, it means that you will not feel food-deprived while asleep. Therefore, make sure you sleep for no fewer than eight hours a day to have a perfect fasting period.

Keep Your Body Hydrated

Fasting for the majority of hours in a day doesn't mean that a dieter should stop drinking water. In fact, it is crucial that you stay hydrated while fasting. It keeps the body's metabolism in good working condition. Staying hydrated will also stave off hunger pangs as liquid takes up room inside the stomach. While practicing intermittent fasting, you can drink herbal tea and other low-calorie drinks as substitutes for water.

Avoid Junk and Processed Foods

Before going into the fasting phase, avoid the temptation to load up on junk, sugary, and processed foods. Instead, eat fresh vegetables and fruits to ensure intake of adequate proteins and fats. Proteins and fats will maintain energy levels in the body. If you eat only a sugar-heavy or carbohydrate-heavy meal, you are more likely to get hungry quicker. For example, a last meal towards the fasting period may include a chicken breast, a piece of garlic bread, and salad made of lettuce, tomatoes, sliced onion, and a vinaigrette dressing.

Incorporate a Tailored Exercising Plan

Exercising during intermittent fasting is optional. It only acts as a catalyst for fast weight loss. If you have to incorporate any exercise plan, tailor it to meet your desired body outcome. For more weight loss, focus on aerobics and cardio-based workouts. Exercising during the fasting phase means that you are performing fasted training. On the other hand, exercising after eating means that you are performing fed training.

Many people find it more viable to exercise after eating. They cite the fact that exercising after a meal gives the body enough energy for working out. In a nutshell, just select a workout schedule that fits your ability.

How to Handle the Inevitable Hunger

Most notably, many people stop following intermittent fasting because they experience hunger pains. However, the inventors of the various different types of intermittent fasting methods believe that there are possible remedies for this. Here are tips on how to handle the inevitable hunger while fasting.

Have the Right Mindset

It is important to develop the right mentality when it comes to intermittent fasting. You won't starve to death from fasting! This is a negative mindset that will just instill fear and cause you to deviate from your original weight loss goal. When you're hungry, convince yourself that you will sail through. After all, the human body has evolved to handle periods of fasting since ancient times.

Have a Snacking Plan

Generally, snacks are meant to lessen hunger pains. They help followers of intermittent fasting to sail through long periods of fasting without eating. If you feel hungry during the fasting period, it is prudent to eat a snack. Make sure you eat a snack that contains a lot of healthy amounts of carbs and fats. Otherwise, eat a piece of fruit. Snacking time should be strategically fixed in the fasting phase.

Balance Your Macronutrients

The macronutrients you need to be most concerned with include proteins, carbs, and fats. Many people fail at intermittent fasting because they go very low on carbs. They are unaware that fasting doesn't require alteration of macronutrients. It is ideal to eat a minimum of 0.6g carbs per body mass combined with twenty-five to thirty percent fats out of your total caloric intake.

Keep Active

The more you stay idle, the more you will develop negative thinking about fasting. In fact, you'll feel hungrier. Do something you enjoy. For example, have a walk in the park while listening to your favorite playlist. This will be helpful since you will lose extra fat. Contrary to the thinking of some dieters, watching TV and spending almost the whole day on social media is the opposite of keeping yourself active. Instead, keep yourself busy while at the same time staying productive.

Get Enough Sleep

Short periods of sleep time are associated with a decrease in leptin and consecutive elevation in ghrelin. This causes more hunger. A study was conducted to determine the effects of sleep patterns on fasting. Findings from the study indicate that better sleep may lead to an increase in weight loss.

How to Manage Eating Out in Restaurants

From time to time, there is a high likelihood that a woman will get an invitation for a meal out. In most situations, it is inevitable. After all, it may be taken as a gesture of lack of gratitude or even as rudeness to turn down an offer by a spouse, close friend, or relative. On the other hand, any woman is financially capable of treating herself to a meal out. This will lead to unplanned eating. It is rare that such a meal will coincide with the scheduled eating time. Thus, intermittent fasting can affect social situations involving eating. Intermittent fasters should know what to do in such situations. Below are tips on how to manage eating in a restaurant.

Don't Eat Your Next Meal

You might not be able to get the same chance to eat out in for quite some time. Knock yourself out! You can eat as much as you want. However, note that you should not eat the next meal on your fasting schedule. This would be improper because you are already full. Moreover, eating the next scheduled meal means you will be breaking the fast, so the overall effect of fasting in that specific day will be negligible. You'll need to fast for a longer window after your spontaneous meal.

Avoid Sugary, Junk, and Processed Foods

A restaurant will have all types of delicacies including all types of junk and processed foods. Don't eat any of them. Having any of these foods will negate the effects of fasting. In fact, some foods, like fries, may contain unhealthy amounts of fats. Additionally, sugary, junk, and processed foods may drastically increase the levels of calories in the body.

Eat Small Amount of Food If You Have To

If the restaurant does not have any food that matches what you want to have, eat a small amount of what they offer. If you are a woman who doesn't like to see food going to waste, share the extra. Even more, you can request that the leftover food be wrapped to-go. Ensure you take a small satiating amount of food.

Order Meals That Conform To Your Customized Meal Plan

Restaurants may not necessarily have meals available for every type of diet. They cater to diversified customer needs by preparing a variety of foods. While eating out, a dieter on intermittent fasting should be choosy on what to eat. Additionally, there are two things that should concern that dieter. First, whether or not it is eating time. Secondly, the number of calories in the available foods. These are two things that may almost be impossible to care about during a meal out. To avoid the worry, ensure you order what seems to conform to the recommended foods. Otherwise, skip the meal and order a low-calorie drink. Do not forget the foods suggested by your dietician!

Chapter Three
Benefits of Intermittent Fasting

Health Benefits of Intermittent Fasting

Fasting is not a new practice. It started a long time ago as a religious undertaking. Unfortunately, our ancestors had to go through fasting periods caused by lack of food. Eventually, it was determined to have dietary benefits. As far back as the 1930s, scientists started exploring the medical benefits of intermittent fasting. Most notably, intermittent fasting is a great way to get lean without going on any diet. People who practice intermittent fasting are able to keep their muscle mass while getting slim. Below is an impressive list of therapeutic benefits that one can get from practicing intermittent fasting.

Enhanced Weight Loss

The main reason for practicing intermittent fasting is to enhance weight loss. In intermittent fasting, one eats fewer meals than usual. This makes it possible to limit the number of calories consumed within a day. Additionally, intermittent fasting has proven to enhance hormone function to accelerate weight loss. Higher levels of norepinephrine (noradrenaline) hormone and reduced insulin levels during intermittent fasting increase the breakdown of body fats and facilitate its use for energy.

For this reason, the metabolic rate increases by up to fifteen percent and the body can burn more calories.

According to a recent scientific study, intermittent fasting can boost weight loss by at least ten percent over three to twenty weeks. This is a considerable amount of weight loss that will lead to achieving the desired body mass. Many women who practice intermittent fasting lost more than eight percent of their waist circumference. This indicates that there is a considerable loss of belly fat, a harmful fat in the abdominal cavity that may cause obesity and other diseases. Even as this is a perfect weight loss technique, it is imperative to note that there is less muscle loss.

Longer Life Span

Scientists have long known that caloric restriction in intermittent fasting is an effective way to increase lifespan. Research was conducted in 1945, where it was discovered that intermittent fasting extends life in mice. Additionally, more research was carried out in human beings and it was found out that alternate-day intermittent fasting leads to longer lifespans. From a logical viewpoint, this makes sense. This is because fasting gives the body's cells the ability to detox and get recycled into the body functions. Therefore, the body can slow down aging and even prevent age-related diseases. People get hesitant when it comes to adopting intermittent fasting to experience this benefit. Who wants to starve themselves in the name of living longer? Even as many people want to live longer, not all of them may seriously engage in fasting. However, many women will starve themselves to gain the desired shape and body size.

Reduced Risk of Cancer

Studies have been done to determine how fasting can prevent cancer and even slow or stop its progression. Findings indicate that fasting can be an effective technique for dealing with cancer. It kills cancer cells while boosting the immune system. Ideally, fasting leads to inadequate nutrients that feed the body cells. In simple words, fasting fights cancer cells by starving them to death. Is it not a good way to fight cancerous cells from propagating in the body?

A recent study suggests that the side effects of chemotherapy may be reduced by fasting. Further information on the same study shows that intermittent fasting supports chemotherapy, resulting in better cure rates and fewer deaths of cancer patients. The extent to which intermittent fasting fights cancer cells is still under study. Scientists intend to obtain a comprehensive analysis of how effective intermittent fasting may become incorporated as a cancer therapy.

Syncing of Circadian Rhythms and Fighting off Metabolic Disease

Circadian rhythm refers to a sleep and wake cycle that is naturally designed to regulate feelings of sleepiness and wakefulness. People with a circadian rhythm disorder often can't sleep comfortably. With intermittent fasting, there is a potential improvement in the body's circadian rhythm. In addition, there is a measurable enhancement of the body's metabolism. Practicing fasting in the evening may be effective in losing weight.

Eating certain foods before bedtime is linked to a weight gain and sleep disturbances. It may also cause acid reflux. Studies have established that fasting can reset the circadian clock and improve these situations. Therefore, you can practice intermittent fasting if you want to improve your circadian rhythms. Combine fasting and going to bed earlier to improve circadian rhythms and fight off metabolic disease.

Lowered Risk for Cardiovascular Disease

Sadly, a large number of people around the world die of heart disease every year. However, the risk of heart disease can be reduced by following a healthy lifestyle. It is simple! Adopt the right eating habits, exercise, quit smoking, and stop excessive alcohol intake. Our major interest in this case is adopting healthy eating habits.

Research has shown that intermittent fasting helps in curtailing cardiovascular diseases. Restricting calories every day leads to glycemic control and insulin resistance. For example, people following the alternate-day fasting regimen successfully lose weight, have reduced blood pressure, and diminish their LDL—"bad" cholesterol. In turn, possibilities of developing cardiovascular disease are drastically reduced.

Lowered Oxidative Stress and Inflammation in the Body

Oxidative stress is a leading cause of many chronic diseases. It involves a damaging reaction of unstable molecules, called free radicals, with other vital molecules like protein and DNA. When such important molecules are damaged, they are of no use in the body. Several studies have shown that intermittent fasting enhances the body's resistance to oxidative stress. Additionally, intermittent fasting can help fight inflammation in the body.

Beneficial to Heart Health

Notably, heart disease is among the world's biggest killers. However, there are various healthy ways of curbing the chances of developing any heart problems. Intermittent fasting reduces numerous health risks associated with heart complications. Such risks include high blood pressure, inflammatory markers, increased blood sugar, and bad cholesterol levels. How does intermittent fasting help in fighting heart-related complications?

Reducing the number of meals translates to reducing calories. The body mechanisms may burn fats and use them in the form of energy. This curtails any potential accumulation of calories and fatty compounds in blood vessels. Due to this, the blood streams throughout the body without any hiccup. The heart's ability to pump blood is not interrupted.

Reduced Risk of Diabetes

Many people have pre-diabetes, including a majority of women. The condition leads to type 2 diabetes within a short period, especially if not treated. Losing weight as a result of intermittent fasting can help in fighting diabetes. How does this happen? When weight is lost, the body becomes more insulin-sensitive. This means that blood sugar levels are lowered and this results in a reduced risk of developing diabetes.

Intermittent fasting helps pre-diabetics by making their bodies produce insulin less often. By skipping meals as a method of intermittent fasting, the body is denied the ability to release more glucose (or sugar compounds) into the bloodstream. When diagnosed with pre-diabetes, one can successfully overcome the problem by adopting intermittent fasting. Additionally, fasting restores insulin secretion and promotes the generation of new-insulin producing pancreatic beta cells.

Boosted Cellular Repair

When fasting, cells begin a cellular detoxification process called autophagy. All the waste products in the cells are removed in the process. The process involves cells collapsing and metabolizing broken and dysfunctional proteins that accumulate inside cells over time. Increased autophagy has been proven to provide protection against several diseases, including cancer and Alzheimer's disease.

Increased Brain Performance

We all want to keep our brain sharp. Intermittent fasting can enhance various metabolic features known to be vital for brain health. Research to prove how intermittent fasting improves brain function has been carried out a number of times. Findings indicate that fasting helps to increase the production of a hormone called brain-derived neurotrophic factor (BDNF) which plays an important role in brain functions. A deficiency of this hormone can lead to depression and various brain problems. Other scientific studies suggest that intermittent fasting prevents short-term memory loss. Additionally, it reduces brain damage and degeneration. Several studies show that intermittent fasting may increase the growth of new nerve cells. This is important for brain development and function.

Chapter Four
The Side Effects

Side Effects of Intermittent Fasting

Even as intermittent fasting may have health benefits, it has drawbacks that may prove detrimental. That is the reason why you should only adopt intermittent fasting under the guidance of an expert. Do not be blinded by the many health benefits and forget to look into the side effects. So, what are the concerns of intermittent fasting?

Infertility

Nutritionists strongly advocate caution for women considering intermittent fasting. This is because it can be dangerous for women. Women engaging in fasting may face problems when trying to conceive. Additionally, intermittent fasting may jeopardize the health of pregnant and breastfeeding women. Adequate caloric and nutrient intake are essential for a healthy reproductive system.

According to doctors, loss of menstrual cycle (amenorrhea) is directly linked to undereating and low body weight. The restrictive nature of intermittent fasting can interfere with fertility and cause low libido. Nutritionists suggest that intermittent fasting is best done by individuals without any stress or energetic demands on the body.

Impaired Athletic Performance

Getting the most out of your workout comes down to carefully replenishing body energy. Restricting calories for a long time can get in the way. If your workout is not timed perfectly during the fasting phase, you could miss out on an important window for muscle growth and glycogen replenishment. This may cause sluggish workout performance. In addition, lack of sufficient glycogen in the body may lead to a breakdown of metabolism which boosts muscle growth.

May Cause Disordered Eating

It may not be officially reported by a majority of dieters, but there is a high tendency to overindulgence during the feast phase. Intermittent fasting gives people the liberty to eat whatever they wish for a short period. By so doing, one may develop bad eating habits trying to eat everything they can within the limited eating time. Actually, complications brought about by overindulgence, like irritable bowel syndrome and abdominal gastric disorder, may become rampant. It may also undo weight loss efforts by a certain percentage, especially if a dieter is fond of eating more calories and fats. Not only will this negate weight loss benefits, but it will also lead to dangerous disorderly binging patterns over time.

Risk of Negative Health Consequences

Some negative health changes may occur due to an unhealthy adoption of intermittent fasting. This makes the body vulnerable to health complications such as sleep problems, changes in menstrual cycles, acne, loss of libido, and headaches among others. Furthermore, beginners of intermittent fasting may suffer from hormonal imbalances. Consequently, this can lead to insomnia, stress, and thyroid problems. Supervision and approval of a physician are necessary to monitor body functions. If not curbed, these health complications can result in chronic diseases.

Malnutrition and Starvation

Depriving the body of necessary nutrients will never be a formula for cultivating ultimate health. Even conventional approaches to dieting suggest that you have to eat enough and follow a healthy diet for enhanced growth and development of the body. It may not seem like a big problem, since intermittent fasting has such a small window for snacking, but snacks don't provide the body with the required nutrients. Malnutrition may have a wide spectrum of consequences that nobody wants to experience.

Adrenals May Get Exhausted

The main role of the adrenals is regulating blood sugar.

Eating anything you want during the feasting phase may cause an abnormal increase of sugar in the body. In turn, controlling the increased levels of sugar may overwork adrenals. Assuming that tired adrenals will regulate blood sugar is the same as asking a tired or unwell woman to prepare a yummy meal. Normal eating patterns do not cause any negative impact on the adrenals. This is because an average amount of sugar is easily regulated by adrenals. In short, eating regularly gives adrenals less work and allows them to repair themselves more quickly.

In addition to the listed side effects, some people attribute the following cons to intermittent fasting.

It is not Realistic for the Long Run

Like most diets, intermittent fasting is not easy to stick to in the long run. A recent study shows that the dropout rate from intermittent fasting is higher than in daily caloric restriction plans. Unfortunately, there are also not enough studies to show the long-term effects of weight loss through intermittent fasting. More studies are underway to help show intermittent fasting can enable weight loss.

May Not be Right for Everyone

We are all different and may not react in a similar manner towards dietary changes. Intermittent fasting is not the best choice for pregnant and lactating mothers. Adolescents shouldn't practice intermittent fasting at all because their body is in a stage that needs high levels of energy. Athletes may experience fatigue, which may alter their interest and strength. The elderly, or people suffering from metabolic diseases such as diabetes and thyroid gland dysfunction, may need to consult a doctor before adopting intermittent fasting.

Why Intermittent Fasting is Not Working

Like many diet plans that are prone to failure, intermittent fasting may not have any impact on a dieter. Common mistakes that can negate the tremendous health benefits of intermittent fasting include overeating or fasting for a negligible period. High discipline is needed to ensure successful intermittent fasting. Otherwise, it will just prove hard to adopt the calorie-downsizing plan. If you are practicing intermittent fasting but not losing weight, you may be doing it wrong! Below are some highlights to enlighten you on what you could be doing wrong.

Failure to Plan

If you don't carefully plan an intermittent fasting schedule, it may well fail. Planning is the key to success, especially for things that dictate strict adherence. Your discipline in maintaining specific fasting patterns may lessen. You may be surprised to find yourself at a party, enjoying all types of delicacies even during the fasting phase. Many dieters think that they can make up late for the ruined fasting phase. That doesn't work. Dieters wanting to try intermittent fasting should understand that consistency is the key to effective weight loss.

Your Fast is Too Short

Unfortunately, many people want to adopt intermittent fasting but are not able to stop eating for a long time. Their stomachs will not stop rumbling and hunger pangs make them uncomfortable the whole day. For this reason, such people find themselves fasting for a negligible period of time. They may end up realizing that the short period of time is all for nothing. If not for nothing, it definitely did not lead to the desired result. Are you among that category of people?

Well, you need a complete overhaul of your fasting schedule to take on board longer fasting periods. It may be hard for beginners. Starting with an eight- to ten-hour fast could serve as a good beginning. Afterward, a longer period should be adopted. Actually, thirteen to fourteen hours is probably the bare minimum for successful intermittent fasting.

You Are Overeating

Many people often justify their bad eating habits during the eating phase of intermittent fasting. They cite the fact that there are no restrictions on any category of foods. However, they do not understand that they may be consuming an excess number of calories. Excess calories may overstay in the body in an unused state even during the fasting. One should eat until satiety. Overeating will ruin the fasting plan. When you're hungry before eating time, you're allowed a snack.

You Are Above Calorie Maintenance

Intermittent fasting is not entirely for calorie management. It is about influencing your natural fat-burning mechanisms through eating patterns. This leads to growth hormone secretion, leptin, ghrelin, insulin sensitivity, and enhanced metabolic rate. However, you can cancel out all of these helpful effects by eating too many calories. By eating any amount of calories as you practice fasting, high levels of calories accumulate in the body. It is imperative to note that a caloric deficit will speed up the process of fat loss.

Your Diet is Defective

It is true that intermittent fasting may not dictate what types of food you do or do not eat. This means that anyone can eat almost everything while during the eating time. Due to this, one may end up ruining the benefits of intermittent fasting. Internet stories and anecdotal evidence of people eating everything while doing intermittent fasting is misleading. Do not rely on eating plans that aren't recommended by doctors or dieticians.

Furthermore, understanding the types of food to eat and those to eat less of or give up completely should be paramount. It is prudent to clean up your diet as much as possible. For instance, you may want to limit sugar, processed foods, fried and fast foods, and refined grains.

You Regularly Break the Fast

Breaking the fasting phase means that you eat before the stipulated time. This negates the impact of the fasting. For those practicing daily intermittent fasting, consuming food before time can wipe out an entire day's worth of fasting. Actually, consuming too many calories may also equate to breaking the fast. Besides, one should be aware of zero-calorie foods, drinks, and condiments. Some of them have a substantial amount of calories. They are just deemed to have zero calories because they are below a certain threshold. When you are not sure whether a drink contains a lot of calories or not, just drink lots of water.

Being Concerned With Negativity

People, especially your friends, relatives, and colleagues, may start discouraging you when you go on a diet. In fact, they will start explaining all the side effects of specific dieting plans like they are nutrition specialists. Do not listen to their advice! Rather, get proper advice from your physician or dietician. It is important to only disclose your fasting plan to people who can give your support and inspire you to perfect it.

Subjecting your mind to thinking about the proven side effects of interment fasting will also affect your devotion to the method as a weight loss remedy. Be focused on what fasting can help you to achieve. After all, not all people feel the side effects associated with intermittent fasting.

You Need To Exercise

If intermittent fasting is not working for you, it may be wise to embrace exercise. The best thing with intermittent fasting is that you can take an exercise break during the fasting phase. It will act as a catalyst for weight loss. Also, it may help in burning excess calories which may impair the efforts of a dieter to lose weight. However, it may not be necessary if you first address the issues listed above.

Weight Loss Maintenance

Research has shown that modern women relentlessly strive to lose weight. The zeal of some has led them to attend gym sessions while others carry out exercises at home. Regardless of where the workout happens, the core aim remains weight loss. Below is an excellent plan that works for every woman.

Be Consistent

Do not quit within the first two days of experiencing hunger pains. It will only take around three days for you to learn to cope with the effects of long periods without foods. Additionally, there are weeks where you may not notice any weight loss. This doesn't mean that the intermittent fasting is ineffective. You should continue to ensure your body adjusts to fasting. Be patient and do not be discouraged.

Eat Healthily

Avoid foods such as cakes, cookies, junk and processed foods, and other unhealthy foods. Sugary and high-fat foods will only make your efforts to lose weight futile. It is prudent to restructure your meals to ensure that the ingredients are low fat, low calorie, and less sugar. Eat more proteins and fiber-rich foods.

Take Calorie Deficit Breaks

You can take a calorie break every two weeks even as you are on intermittent fasting. This means going with a diet that has zero or negligible amounts of calories for an entire day. For example, boiled yams with fermented milk (with no sugar) at lunch and spaghetti with half a glass of milk for dinner. Caloric deficit breaks result in more weight loss. This method of dieting helps to keep the body from slowing down, allowing you to burn more calories.

Eventually, you will lose a measurable amount of body mass within a few weeks.

Get Enough Sleep

Most people sleep for no less than six hours per night, which qualifies as enough sleep. Getting enough sleep keeps stress under control. Stress is one of the factors that tend to slow the process of losing weight. This is because sleep deprivation and an increase of stress hormones in the body raise blood sugar levels. In turn, this slows weight loss by increasing calories in the body.

Adopt Some Exercises

As you may have noted, exercising during the fasting period is optional. Combining exercise with fasting enhances faster weight loss. It helps to raise the rate of weight loss by burning more fat in the body. Any weight loss plan for women may be hard. This is because women have brittle and soft bodies which may take some time to get used to exercise. Do not give up easily!

Thoughts and Misconceptions about Intermittent Fasting

Like any other well-known dieting plans that have immense positive health effects, intermittent fasting has garnered a number of biased and baseless misconceptions. Most of the misconceptions are about the ramifications.

As it is, people cannot stop circulating information about fasting on the internet, whether positive or negative. This is a clear indication that intermittent fasting is indeed a force to be reckoned with when it comes to dieting. This part aims at separating truth from fiction. Below are some common fallacies about fasting and the corresponding truth.

You Can Eat All You Want During a Single Eating Phase

Some dieters think that they can eat all they want during the eating window. This is totally erroneous and misinformed. Typically, the phrase "eat all you can" may translate to overeating. Mind you, overeating has major drawbacks for weight loss goals. Eating all you want is not appropriate and can negate the effects of fasting in an entire day. For instance, overeating may put you over recommended caloric levels. Just eat what will give you satiety. Additionally, tracking the number of macronutrients you eat is vital for successful fasting.

You Should Fast More When Fat Loss Stalls

Why should you eat more to reignite weigh loss? Won't that make you gain weight? It is true that a dieter may not witness any weight loss at some time. There is information in another section of this book on why fasting may not be working for a dieter. Fasting for longer periods of time can be harmful to your health. Actually, it can lead to starvation which may have a serious negative effect on a dieter's metabolism. Therefore, more fasting will not help if you are eating too much and not tracking calories and macronutrients.

You Cannot Practice Fasted Exercise

Misleading information suggests that a dieter cannot perform fasted exercising. As stated earlier, exercising can enhance the impact of intermittent fasting. Exercising while you are fasting is helpful in ensuring burning off excess calories. You may even forget you're hungry. As long as you have enough sleep and get adequate rest, fasted exercise should not be detrimental for you. Nonetheless, this does not mean that fasted exercise is for everyone. Some people may feel dizzy and lack the energy to keep up. That is not an alarming disability. It is normal.

You Can Ignore Tracking Macros

Tracking macros is not only specific to intermittent fasting. Most diet plans advocate the monitoring of macros. The biggest mistake that a follower of intermittent fasting may commit is to abstain from tracking macros. Eating any macros and having the mentality of "eating whatever you like" will only reduce the benefits of fasting. Even though you may increase the fasting period, nothing will be achieved without proper dieting. It is important to note that you must track and make proper adjustments to macros while fasting. Another aspect of tracking is in the progress you are making within a given period. From one week to another, carefully track your weight loss.

Note that these are only a few examples of misconceptions about intermittent fasting. If you come across information concerning fasting that you are not sure about, consult your dietician.

Chapter Five
Examples of Recipes with Nutrition and Calorie Information

SNACK RECIPES

Broccoli with garlic and lemon

Number of servings: 2

Ingredients

- 4 cups broccoli florets
- 1 teaspoon olive oil
- 1 tablespoon minced garlic
- 1 teaspoon lemon zest
- 1/4 teaspoon kosher salt
- 1/4 teaspoon ground black pepper

Instructions

1. Boil 1 cup of water in a small saucepan.
2. Add the broccoli to the boiling water and cook until tender.
3. Drain broccoli.
4. Heat the oil in a small sauté pan over medium-high.
5. Add the garlic and fry for just 30 seconds then add lemon zest, broccoli, salt and pepper.
6. Mix thoroughly and serve.

Nutritional Information per Serving

Serving Amount: 1 cup

Calories	45	Protein	3g
Cholesterol	0mg	Dietary fiber	3g
Monounsaturated fat	1g	Sodium	153mg
Trans fat	0g	Total sugar	2g
Total fat	1g	Total carbohydrates	7g

Green beans with red pepper and garlic

Number of servings: 6

Ingredients

- 1-pound green beans, stems trimmed
- 2 teaspoons olive oil
- 1 red bell pepper, seeded and cut into thin slices
- 1/2 teaspoon chili paste or red pepper flakes
- 1 clove garlic, finely chopped
- 1 teaspoon sesame oil
- 1/2 teaspoon salt

- 1/4 teaspoon freshly ground black pepper

Instructions

1. Cut the beans into 2-inch slices.
2. Add water to a large saucepan until 3/4 full and boil.
3. Now, add the beans and cook until they turn bright green and are tender-crunchy.
4. Drain the beans and immerse them in a bowl of ice water. Drain again and put aside.
5. Heat the olive oil over medium heat in a large frying pan and add the bell pepper. Toss and stir for about 1 minute.
6. Add beans and fry for 1 more minute.
7. Add chili paste and garlic and stir for 1 minute.
8. After the beans become tender and bright green, sprinkle with the sesame oil and season with the salt and pepper.
9. Serve while hot.

Nutritional Information per Serving

Serving Amount: 3/4 cup

Calories	54	Sodium	202mg
Cholesterol	0mg	Protein	2g

Dietary fiber	2g	Monounsaturated fat	1g
Total fat	2g	Added sugars	0g
Trans fat	0g	Total carbohydrate	7g

LUNCH RECIPES

Avocado deviled eggs

Number of Servings: 6

Ingredients

- 6 eggs, hard boiled
- 1 ripe avocado, peeled and pitted
- 1 1/2 teaspoons lime juice
- 3 tablespoons light mayonnaise
- 1 teaspoon chopped parsley
- 1 teaspoons ground cayenne pepper
- 1 clove fresh garlic, minced

Instructions

1. Cut all the eggs lengthwise. Remove the yolks and set aside.
2. In a medium-sized bowl, combine the egg yolks, half of the parsley, cayenne pepper mayonnaise, avocado, lime juice, and garlic.
3. Scoop the mixture into the egg whites and decorate with the rest of the chopped parsley.
4. Serve immediately

Nutritional Information per Serving

Serving Amount: 2 half portions

Calories	97	Sodium	126mg
Total fat	7g	Dietary fiber	2g
Saturated fat	1.5g	Total carbohydrates	3.5g
Monounsaturated fat	4g	Added sugars	0g
Cholesterol	93mg	Protein	5g

Spinach dip with mushrooms

Number of Servings: 10

Ingredients

- 1 package (10 ounces) frozen chopped spinach (thawed and squeezed dry)
- 1 1/2 cups fat-free sour cream
- 1 cup fat-free mayonnaise
- 1 cup chopped fresh mushrooms
- 3 green onions, chopped

Instructions

1. Mix all the ingredients in a medium-sized bowl.
2. Blend well, cover, and put in a freezer for around 10-15 minutes.
3. Serve frozen with a variety of raw vegetables.

Nutritional Information per Serving

Serving Amount: Half cup

Calories	56	Protein	3g
Cholesterol	3mg	Sodium	268mg
Trans fat	0g	Total carbohydrates	11g
Dietary fiber	1g	Total sugars	2g
Monounsaturated fat	0g		

DINNER RECIPES

Pita pizza

Number of servings: 2

Ingredients

- 2 whole-wheat pita loaves
- 1/2 cup marinara
- 1/2 cup diced red onion
- 1/4 cup sliced button mushrooms
- 1/4 cup diced pineapple
- 1/4 cup diced bell pepper
- 6 tablespoons part-skim mozzarella cheese
- 1/4 cup reduced-fat feta cheese
- 2 teaspoons turkey bacon bits

Instructions

1. Heat the oven to 190 C (375F).
2. Lightly coat a baking sheet using some cooking spray.
3. Put the pitas on the baking sheet and spread the marinara over them.
4. Cover the pizzas with equal amounts of onion, pineapple, peppers, and mushrooms and sprinkle with cheeses and bacon bits.
5. Bake until all the cheese is golden brown in color.
6. Remove from the oven and serve.

Nutritional Information per Serving

Serving Amount: 1 pizza

Calories	324	Sodium	820mg
Total fat	17g	Protein	17g
Monounsaturated fat	1g	Total carbohydrates	48g
Cholesterol	21mg	Total sugars	9g
Saturated fat	3g	Dietary fiber	4g

Rice noodles with spring vegetables

Number of servings: 6

Ingredients

- 1 package rice noodles
- 1 tablespoon peanut oil
- 1 tablespoon sesame oil
- 1 tablespoon grated fresh ginger
- 2 garlic cloves finely chopped
- 2 tablespoons low-sodium soy sauce
- 1 cup small broccoli florets
- 1 cup fresh bean sprouts

- 8 cherry tomatoes, halved
- 1 cup chopped fresh spinach
- 1 scallions, chopped
- Crushed red chili flakes (optional)

Instructions

1. Fill a relatively large pot 3/4 full with water and boil it.
2. Add the noodles and cook for around 5-6 minutes or according to the package instructions.
3. Remove and rinse the noodles with cold water and set aside.
4. In another frying pan, heat oils over moderate heat and add ginger and garlic. Stir while frying.
5. Add and stir the soy sauce and broccoli and carry on cooking for about 4 minutes. Add the remaining veggies and cooked noodles and toss until warmed.
6. Divide the noodles among warmed plates and cover each with crushed red chili flakes (optional).
7. Serve while hot.

Nutritional Information per Serving

Serving Amount: 1 1/2 cups

Calories	205	Sodium	215mg
Cholesterol	0mg	Dietary fiber	1g
Total carbohydrates	37g	Total fat	5g
Saturated fat	1g	Added sugars	0g
Monounsaturated fat	2g	Protein	3g